Emotional Psychology

*Skills, Tricks, and Techniques to Improve
Your Self-Esteem, Eliminate the Power to
Negative Emotions, Build Self-Confidence and
Find Long-Lasting Success*

Description

Is it true that you are worn out on advancing toward the back of the class since you are excessively frightened, making it impossible to demonstrate your venture, despite the fact that you know it is superior to anything everybody else's? Is it accurate to say that you are tired of continually being imperceptible because of every one of your companions who appear to have far more energy in their progression? Do you battle to reveal to yourself everything is okay and that you are amazing while at the same time preparing before the mirror? Does strolling over the limit of your entryway panic the living crap out of you; will be you apprehensive how everyone around you will see you? Assuming any of these inquiries relate to you, at that point you have unearthed quite recently the perfect place! You, old buddy, are unfortunately and significantly ailing in certainty and we have to settle this!

The contents of this book include:

- *Why our world is inevitably full of Debbie-Downers and those that just can't seem to get their chins up*

- *Simple and easy ways to reduce stress in your life that will lift that heavy boulder off your shoulder*

- *How to live in a brighter and more positive light on a daily basis*

- *A few great ways to get yourself to relax in order to really take a deeper, more intricate look at your life*

- *Many ways that you can build up your self-confidence and self-esteem to live a better life!*

- *And more!*

My kindred pursuer, on the off chance that you have gone over the portrayal of this book, more than likely you are as of now searching for approaches to feel better about yourself! Why not give this book a shot and see the enchantment that it can work appropriate inside your everyday life in giving you another standpoint? Truly, what do you need to lose? Is it true that it isn't the ideal opportunity for a change of pace? Aren't you prepared to bring on the day with a solid and forceful certainty? Wouldn't it feel decent to disregard the contemplations of others and stay gently inside your own particular minimal world? At that point give the substance of these sections a shot to enable you to out! With a little know-how and information, a man can change in a variety of angles. What's more, you will perceive how simply the subject of certainty can change a man for whatever is left of their life. Trust me on this one.

In the event that you are going for the buy this book now, good fortunes! On the off chance that you are quite recently simply contemplating what is within this book, truly give your life a look over and think about what you have to lose. With increasing fearlessness, only great things! On the off chance that you need to change your life, you need to have confidence and begin making starting strides in the correct footing. This book is an extraordinary beginning in doing just that!

Table of Contents

Introduction

Congratulations on purchasing your very own copy of *Emotional Psychology*. Thank you so much for doing so.

The accompanying parts will talk about a portion of the ways that you can fuse in your own particular day by day life that will lead you on a way to a more cheerful sure self! A longing to be sure and more positive on the planet we live in today is a quality that practically each and every individual on this planet pines for. Getting to be and really being more joyful in your skin is in no way, shape or form a simple deed to maintain.

You will find how critical being certain is inside numerous parts of your life and how you can advance a couple of ventures beyond with the tips that are concealed inside these sections. Getting to be plainly certain will lead you to general achievement when you can at long last free yourself from the dim mists that dependably appear to be approaching over you! You will likewise discover that you are in no way, shape or form alone with regards to having an absence of certainty. A significant number of us encounter this and it cuts down our soul as well as our capability to be as well as can be expected conceivably be.

The last section will investigate how to leap effectively over obstructions that will unavoidably come toward you all through life. Regardless of how sure you feel, circumstances happen that push us to the brink of collapse, making us feel anything besides sure. We should talk about that it is so essential to ascend go down and battle and how to restore that certainty and confidence that you worked so darn hard to accomplish!

There are plenty of books about polishing up your personal well-being on the market, thanks again for choosing this one! Every effort was made to ensure it is full of as much useful information as possible. Please enjoy!

Why a Lower Sense of Self is More Prevalent than Ever Before

On the off chance that you are perusing this book, you are more than likely an individual searching for direction about how to wind up plainly more sure and confident, your identity and your identity getting to be. We have all been at places throughout our lives when we are far not as much as prepared to confront deterrents when individuals cut us so far down that we have not one piece of information how to bring ourselves move down for air.

Instabilities are simply the hidden center of our absence of self-assurance. Actually, as a general rule, we feel truly doltish for our tensions that we have about our general surroundings. Every last individual has no less than one thing they are shaky about in their own life, regardless of what level it might be on. This is absolutely typical and is a piece of being a normal human. Be that as it may, there are a few people that convey expansive rocks of frailties upon their shoulders each day.

To really get a handle on the comprehension of how a few people can turn out to be so self-assured, it is critical to take a gander at the reasons why we as individuals have a tendency to get tossed underneath the rubble apprehensiveness.

Low confidence – As people, we are our own particular most exceedingly bad commentators. We know the majority of our blemishes and see them just as negative parts of ourselves. We are truly incognizant in regards to our abilities and the special things that one of a kind and wonderful. This just not makes us amazingly envious of everyone around us however it specifically puts fuel on our flames of instability. This prompts a low feeling of self and confidence. Rather than attempting to check why we feel so contrarily towards ourselves, we are stuck of self-indulgence and disgrace for our identity.

Projection – Turn back your brain science books to Sigmund Freud's discoveries and you will discover the projection guideline. This is a mental marvel that goes about as a barrier component by ousting our own instabilities upon another in ways you would like to receive some good feeling or inspiration in return. When you feel or say something negative in regards to another person, particularly certain attributes, as a general rule you are truly discussing yourself.

We let the past characterize us – There are specific encounters that fuel our aversion we have towards ourselves. There can be numerous angles that are in charge of why we feel the way we do about ourselves. Past dismissals, surrender, treacheries or terrible adolescence/youthful adulthood encounters would all be able to be triggers for negative feelings.

To have the capacity to roll out an improvement, one should have the capacity to first perceive the things that they do all the time to put themselves always in the canal. At exactly that point will they have the ability to have the capacity to change their standpoint about themselves and mirror a more constructive light onto other individuals. We are all shaky to some degree, even those that sparkle brilliantly with beyond any doubt sort of certainty. In any case, there are a few signs that a large number of us ourselves to do see as negative until the point when they are brought up. The following are a few things that shaky individuals manage without ever truly acknowledging it. The time has come to call attention to your defects. Sorry, not too bad!

Surrendering effortlessly – The general population who have the greatest issues in settling on choices of where they need their life ways to go are those that surrender effectively while endeavoring new things or simply don't have the energy or craving to make enough of an effort. To have the capacity to carry on with the best life you can, you should fan out and attempt new things with the best endeavors that you got. You live, you learn. Yet, for those lacking fearlessness, they feel they are not equipped for doing such things and remain inside their wellbeing net, failing to reach out for anything beneficial or new.

The consistent dread of judgment – The more uncertain a man is, the additional time their instabilities and the way they feel about themselves abide inside their psyches. These people live in an endless kind of dread and expectation energetically that nobody will see how "defective" they truly are. As mankind, each and every one of us gets a kick out of the chance to think we are not judging, but rather we are. It is something we do consequently. In any case, that shouldn't be the worry. You ought to be asking yourself for what reason it is important what others consider you to such an extent? Many don't think about your defects that you consider all the time in any case.

Maintain a strategic distance from connection with new individuals – Other individuals assume enormous parts in our day by day lives, regardless of whether we get a kick out of the chance to let it out or not. Collaboration with other individuals is a vital component to molding our lives, yet not really generally advantageous. A few of us get included with terrible individuals while others discover their place inside a specialty of sound individuals. Shaky individuals have a tendency to have individuals in their lives that truly don't serve their best enthusiasm for the long run. Being unreliable implies that we normally agree to specific things, including individuals. They are frightened to stretch out and meet anybody new, regardless of the possibility that they know where it counts that those new faces could do them an extraordinary measure of good.

They trust they are sufficiently bad – People with large amounts of instability have a tendency to be those that worthless their way through life. They never attempt to give something on the grounds that they genuinely believe that their "all" is never adequate. The thing is life IS the thing that you put into it. The more, the better for this situation. The less you attempt, the less significance your life will have. Make an existence that merits thinking back on.

Continually keeping down – Those that hold numerous weaknesses within them all the time tend to put the majority of their time and vitality into professing to be individuals they are definitely not. They shroud their imperfections behind an affectation around others. This is an awful quality of life since you will dependably be closing individuals who wish to know the genuine you out. You think the genuine you are disturbing and you don't need it to appear when truly there are most likely many individuals searching for somebody in their life simply like you!

The misguided feeling of self all day, every day – Thanks to weaknesses controlling over your considerations about existence and yourself, these individuals may never truly comprehend what all they are able and who they could move toward becoming in the event that they unshackled themselves from the chains of unconfidence. In the event that one is never legit to whatever is left of the world about who they truly are, we will never discover the spots that we really have a place in our life.

Live in steady dissent – The truth of the matter is nobody is great. Not one single individual on this planet is. So why do we endeavor so frightfully hard for flawlessness? We have to recollect that a few things throughout our life are totally out of our control. Instabilities attempt to disclose to you that you are sufficiently bad and you suck as a man when truly you are great in your own remarkable way! You are tolerating the untruths that your uncertainties are gushing out to you as your reality. Also, that is an unacceptable quality of life.

Passing up a major opportunity for terrific open doors – Each one of us just gets one life to live and tragically, a significant number of us are not living it without limitations at all. Not being certain and submitting to the guidelines that your frailties have laid out for you is truly compelling you to live less. You stress increasingly and live less as your negative musings gather. There are numerous open doors that are sitting tight for your nearness, you simply need to pick not to live by your weaknesses, but rather, change your attitude and grasp the energy of you.

Fizzled connections – Relationships flourish from genuineness and uprightness between two individuals. The main way any sort of relationship can be 100% fruitful is whether you are straightforward with yourself first. Regardless of the amount you attempt to conceal your actual self behind a cover you made, your real nature will inevitably leak out for other individuals you are drawing near with to see. Uncertainties just purpose strains to rise and in productive connections, there is no space for them to live. Shaky individuals regularly flop hopelessly at tolerating their blemishes and grasping them, which in the end prompts the finish of connections and kinships. This is a discouraging truth however unless you change it, you will always be in the example of shocking associations with others. It is imperative to take a shot at yourself first!

In this day and age, it is getting to be plainly less demanding to fall into the traps of uncertainties. Much appreciated the perpetually developing nearness of online networking, we continually are in rivalry against the lives of other individuals. Desire, envy, and lament over your own life energize the uncertainties that we as a whole normally have, causing pressure in your life. It has turned out to be considerably simpler to judge individuals in light of looks, status and what they claim or don't have. We have turned into a general public of things as opposed to positive emotions and activities. Being unconfident is like different feelings that we hate feeling and living through. Much the same as misery, outrage, envy, and so forth, we should recall that it is alright to feel the way we do some of the time, yet that it unfortunate to stay in an especially negative feeling for a really long time. Relies on upon the movements of life, we should feel the way we do now and again to assemble the encounters in life that we have to develop. The rest of this book will illuminate you of approaches to wind up noticeably a more certain person! Good fortunes in finding the certainty that can battle your weaknesses that are within you.

How to Build Your Self-Confidence

Regardless of whether you are as of now a truly gallant individual or you know darn well that you have to chip away at this piece of your own self, this section holds numerous thoughts and tips to help you out in finding that confident form of yourself, or at any rate keeping that piece of you conditioned and prepared forever's sudden impediments. While winding up plainly more certainty is achievable, one must remember that you should have an engaged assurance to better yourself in this office. Picking up the certainty you need to talk to others or attempt new things is in no way, shape or form going to mystically occur without any forethought. The ways that you construct you certainly will likewise saturate how fruitful you can be at accomplishing whatever you set your psyche to. Making an intense certainty is something you ought to be glad for and when you accomplish it you should take sufficient care of it, for it is a critical piece of your identity!

Inside this part, you will run over some really straightforward exhortation that may appear to be inconsequential when you quite recently skim through it. Be that as it may, I guarantee you, on the off chance that you set aside the opportunity to start fusing some of these approaches to manufacture your certainty all the time, you will see real change about how you feel about yourself, others and the obscure. Indeed, even the best of pioneers need certainty and regard every once in a while. It is not a measurement. It is an outlook that takes commitment to keep up, particularly when you get yourself into an unpleasant time. Gratefully, certainty can be educated, rehearsed, accomplished and aced. Consider it an aptitude instead of only an advantage. The rest of this part is brimming with truckloads of approaches to advance your own particular fearlessness. Your welcome!

Introduce Yourself with Confidence

In the event that you are continually chilling on the sofa at home with family or companions, what you look like most likely does not make a difference close as much to you as though you are going to go meet new individuals or give a major discourse. In new circumstances, numerous parts of certainty are stemmed specifically from your appearance. That sounds shallow, however, it is valid. Guaranteeing that you look positive attitude make feel great vibes that will get you through the anxiety of the obscure. When you know and genuinely feel you look great, it appears! Your non-verbal communication is a consistent exhibit of self-assuredness or outrageous weakness. Continuously attempt to introduce yourself in ways that make you look as though you are the face of a circumstance. On the off chance that you look certain, you will feel sure and have the capacity enough to act the part that you need to accomplish.

- *Dress pleasantly* – When you dress pleasantly, it makes a vibe that makes you feel relentless and that you can handle anything that life tosses your direction. This can mean diverse things to every individual. This does not intend to go discharge your financial balance on various new pieces of attire. Yet, when you like the way you look, it is significantly less demanding to introduce yourself in a sure way.

- *Work on positive non-verbal communication* – If you have a tendency to sit slumped over in a seat or stroll with your eyes skimming the floor, it will make you look exceptionally unconfident. Rather, regardless of the circumstance, sit up tall with your shoulders back, hold your head up, grin and look at individuals without flinching while collaborating with them. Work on a firm handshake as well. This will enable you to seem positive about your walk.

- *Speak with confidence* – If you have never been in a swarm that is occupied with an open speaker, go to one. Be aware of the way they convey their addresses to the group. Stupendous speakers that have any kind of effect in those going to talk with relentless, musical and sure tone. Rather than utilizing "ahs" and "uhms" amid stops, they use these breaks in discourse to underscore the thoughts they are attempting to get out. Figuring out how to talk in a confident way will enable your confidence to rise. Individuals will tune into those that go about as their own pioneers and when they see self-assurance transmitting from you as your talk.

- *Think and act in a positive way* – Displaying a positive vitality normally prompts great results much of the time. Indeed, even in the dimmest of conditions, attempt to make the decision to the "I can do it" mentality and abstain from conversing with yourself adversely. Trust me, a stone will be lifted just from being around individuals who genuinely appreciate your conversation. Figure out how to advise when the time has come to put space amongst you and negative impacts, grin increasingly and giggle frequently. Write in an appreciation diary every prior night bed or make this movement a piece of your morning schedule. This helps with recollecting the high purposes of your day/week and also what you have effectively expert. When you are agiler in your appreciation, it will enable you to build up a feeling of peace which specifically fills fearlessness.

Make a move

There is considerably more behind the drapery of the play of certainty than simply your appearance. You should really follow up on the part. Acknowledge things you would typically dodge or reject. Stroll up and cooperate with outsiders at occasions. When you hone straightforward strides to certainty, it will turn out to be second nature to you after some time.

Be Prepared

While there is no correct approach to be set up for everything without exception, you can, in any event, make an endeavor to have some kind of go down arrangement or if nothing else a guide of moves to make when things get somewhat chaotic. Keep in mind this imperative tongue twister: "Earlier arranging anticipates poor execution." The better set we up are for the unavoidably obscure, the more certain we will feel in our competency. Sufficient planning will enable you to abstain from getting thumped over by unforeseen occasions. The more you know the happier you will be. Get the hang of all that you can about the specific range of your profession. Wind up plainly mindful of what drives you to succeed. Plan out objectives and how you envision yourself accomplishing them.

Learn constantly

The lovely thing about our enormous, wide planet and the multifaceted nature of the human personality is that there is never a lot to learn or insufficient space to develop. The more information you procure, the more your fearlessness will be encouraged and you will have the activity to go out and encounter new things, as well as advise other individuals about what you have realized and how you have developed into a superior individual with a more profound understanding as a result of it. Sign yourself up for new classes. Expand your viewpoints on subjects you think you are as of now a specialist at. Odds are you have not exactly turned out to be 100% aced at what you think you have. On the off chance that you had effectively done completely everything in life (which is outlandish, incidentally) at that point that startling feeling that dwells in your trunk would not exist. Grasp the obscure and that frightened sensation. It implies you are going some place new!

Concentrate on creating aptitudes that will advance you beyond in the session of life. Win at things that matter to you. What sort of learning might you be able to gain that could enhance your odds at winning in your own life?

Be Attentive to the Needs of Others

Here and there we fuel our own particular negative contemplations simply by getting to be plainly latched onto our subconscious mind for a really long time. We have a tendency to harp on negative parts of our lives and figure out how to consider our remorseful sentiments of things we have no influence over or can, not anymore change. Rather, hit up a companion or relative and inquire as to whether there is anything you can accomplish for them as opposed to being tied up in your own pool of musings.

Make sure to furnish others with compliments at whatever point you can or make your own particular chances to bring others up. They, as well, are battling with certainty the same amount of as you seem to be, regardless of the possibility that they pass on heaps of it. Guarantee that you are not always doling out a group of tricky types of sweet talk. Individuals will have the capacity to tell on the off chance that you are being genuine or not. Continuously be straightforward with the compliments you give, for they will give the most warmth to other people who get them. Furthermore, as a general rule, the more you give, the more you will in the long run get. Great karma has a decent method for returning to reimburse those that compensation others.

Same goes for your requirements too. Never be hesitant to request offer assistance. It is a major startling world out there! We are not fit for doing everything all alone. Once in a while, it takes limits of fearlessness to just request help.

Spread Your Wings

Regardless of whether you are welcomed by a companion or relative to an occasion or another event, rather than giving out an IOU, extend your points of view and go to! You may never know who you will get the chance to meet and chat with, or what new data you will eat up that could possibly lead you in an alternate way in life. On the off chance that you are somewhat anxious, concentrate on being a useful hand to individuals as opposed to being encompassed by the considerations of what other individuals might be pondering you. Next time you have the inclination you may talk yourself out of going some place, let yourself know "Why not?" and compel yourself into going. As a general rule, you will be happy that you did.

Ensure you are giving yourself bottomless open doors. Attempt another way as opposed to adhering to what you know or what others in your life need you to live next to. DO YOU. The most voyaged ways of life can turn out to be familiar to the point that you will, in the end, wind up plainly detached from life out and out, which in no way, shape or form raises up your regard levels.

What Truly Matters to You?

Getting a handle on a completely clear picture of what you need out of life is one of the principal great strides in arranging your life into picking up a superior feeling of confidence. This can incorporate vocation, individuals, things, parts of life, and so on. On the off chance that you have not yet accomplished what you envision in your psyche all the time, discover roads to get it going! Make a rundown of things that you need to keep in your life, things that you just simply endure in light of the fact that you "need to" and things you need to include for the improvement of your general satisfaction. At that point make a rundown of how to dispose of the negative and recover the positive.

Welcome the Good and the Bad
Life is not all butterflies and rainbows. Perceive the need to recognize that you will go over both astonishing and important circumstances while also encountering unpleasant circumstances that you simply wish to overlook. Regardless, every last circumstance we survive encourages us to develop into the general population we are today. Nobody is invulnerable to awful circumstances. Try not to cover up or be embarrassed about the awful things that have transpired.

Both your qualities and shortcomings ought to be viewed as resources rather than "great" or "terrible" qualities. Qualities can enable you to conquer whatever shortcomings you have. Try not to let what makes you weak undermine your esteem and levels of certainty.

You Deserve Better and Can BE Better
There will be conditions and individuals that will just persistently push your catches until the point that you need to step your foot down and say NO MORE. I merit better! Prepare to be blown away. You are correct. In any case, you more than likely can be better too. You commonly draw in what you are. On the off chance that you are a bubbly, constructive individual, those sorts of individuals and openings will come your direction!

Trust Yourself

There is no inclination more beyond any doubt than what our instinct or our guts let us know. In the event that your intuition breaks out its notice sign, don't disregard it. You were conceived with impulses and hunches which are as it should be. Regardless of the possibility that you are not absolutely certain about yourself, be positive about what your spirit it endeavoring to get crosswise over to you.

Use Fear

Dread has an amusing method for demonstrating to us the approach. It generally appears to summon up circumstances we would have generally not stood up to all alone. It tells us that we can extend our capacities and develop from numerous points of view. Utilize dread further bolstering your good fortune as opposed to giving it a chance to take you over. Give it a chance to enable you to advance.

Quit Comparing Yourself to Others

Our general public does this now like never before. We are continually noiselessly passing judgment on each other, both outsiders and those we cherish alike, once in a while without acknowledging we are doing as such. Try not to endeavor to discover the approval you require through the examination of other individuals.

Self-esteem is not needy

Your inward joy ought not to be managed by the energy of someone else. This is the place many individuals turn out badly seeing someone. They have avoided the progression of chipping away at themselves and finding their own particular joy first and accordingly, rely on upon the nearness of being with someone else to fuel this void piece of their lives. Over the long haul, it won't work out. You can't pour anything from an unfilled pot. You should fill the pot (you) with satisfaction to have the capacity to give out what other individuals require from you.

Make a Positive Environment

The things and individuals that encompass you unreasonably affect your impression of yourself. Arrange your workspace as opposed to being encompassed by a mess. Dispose of negative impacts throughout your life that bring you down as opposed to pulling up. While cleaning up your work area is considerably simpler than saying bye to those in your life that you are in an ideal situation without, both make you feel very elevated.

Channel Your Heroes

Contemplate through the occasions of your life and recollect to somebody you respect and acknowledge for their own particular limits of certainty. Consider what that individual would do or say despite your inconveniences. Figure out how to channel their certainty directly into your own particular life. Envision you have the certainty and confidence of these individuals in new circumstances. Don't really duplicate the methods for these people, however, figure out how to distinguish how they pass on their certainty and endeavor to make sense of constructive, momentous ways that you can imagine a similar sort of confidence.

Acknowledge your Imperfections and Disapproval

Compulsiveness is not feasible, despite the fact that many invest significant energy and hard earned cash endeavoring to accomplish it. As opposed to endeavoring to be immaculate, attempt just to be the best individual you can be. Acknowledge that you will dependably have things to survive and develop from. Embracing this mentality takes into account all that could possibly be needed sufficient space for you to develop as a man. Your life proverb ought to be about improving the best!

Regardless of the amount you endeavor to be your best, there is continually going to be people who object to your life and your choices. Prepare to have your mind blown. They are squandering their profitable time since it is not their life to live, it is your life. You will never have the ability to please completely everybody you gone over in your life, regardless of how hard you attempt. Attempt to make an adjustment that leads you not wind up plainly subject to the endorsement of others. This will lead you to give up your objectives and yearnings. You are basically slighting yourself and this will prompt a noteworthy drop in self-assurance.

Venture Out of Your Comfort Zone

You will never develop and neither will your levels of certainty unless you get yourself out from under that warm cover of recognition and grasp the obscure. Regardless of how tentative you typically are, find that vitality somewhere inside you to talk up amid critical circumstances. Make an arrangement in your mind for the thoughts you wish to examine with others. The more your voice is heard, the more open doors you could have the likelihood of getting your hands on.

Be Humble, Kind and Generous

Despite the fact that this may not appear as though is has anything to do with your certainty, it is an extraordinary bit of its center in all actuality. Being liberal of yourself implies furnishing yourself with the sufficient time to accomplish the things you need to fulfill. This not just goes for dealing with yourself either. Keep in mind that great old Golden Rule that we learned as children? It is something that is as yet a thing however not utilized almost enough in our general public today. When you start to feel better about yourself, you will then have the capacity to extend your positive sentiments onto others and treat them the way you might want to be dealt with.

This will do wonders for your confidence levels. Helping others in helping them feeling cooperative attitude improve you feel limits in a matter of seconds.

Change One Habit at a Time

Every one of us has propensities that we perform regularly that we are not all that glad for. Rather than feeling the need to live next to our propensities and enabling them to constrain us to feel adverse about ourselves, why not make a move to transform one propensity at any given moment? Wake up prior so you have more opportunity to appreciate the morning before work. Smoke one cigarette less a day. Drink a glass of water when you rise. Whatever propensity you need to change or fuse, do it regularly for a month and it will turn out to be second nature. Certain propensities, for instance, flossing your teeth each time you brush, prompts a superior projection of appearance and are little venturing stones in working up your self-assurance.

Concentrate on what YOU Want

In the present society, we are so damn occupied that we truly lose our feeling of self. We overlook what our objectives are and progressed toward becoming too distracted by every other person's life and contrasting our existence with others that we overlook that we are squandering valuable time! What you concentrate on at first opens up your world. When we concentrate on things that make us restless, we thus, are on edge. Rather, invest your energy offering regard for things that move and enable you. Rather than frightening yourself into not accomplishing something you need to accomplish in light of the fact that you are harping on what you would prefer not to happen, consider rather what you might want to happen.

Reduce Stress
through Simplifying your Life

Distinguish Stressors
The initial phase in improving your life is to make note of the things that make you wind up plainly worried in any case. Make a rundown of these specific things so you comprehend what should be chipped away at or completely wiped out keeping in mind the end goal to make more peace inside your day by day life.

De-mess
Your own condition that you harp in every day is an immediate impression of the center parts of your internal being. Everything that you let encompass you conveys to light what brings you either peace or trouble. While the procedure of legitimately de-jumbling is not fast or simple one, you will get yourself more settled for the duration of the day when you can concentrate on more than the things that expend your life. It will likewise hinder you from losing vital articles, similar to auto keys, that can make one restless when they are as of now running late and can't find them.

Many individuals observe cleaning, by and large, to be distressing. I think that it's mitigating. I have an inclination that I am disposing of garbage that I don't need in my life out with the goal that I can prepare for things that better suit my life and where I need to go. Try not to think de-jumbling your life is just about lifeless protests either. Consider people who are a major part of your life now that make you feel adverse or convey harmful sentiments to the surface. You don't need to essentially cut all ties with these specific individuals, however, figure out how to remove yourself. They don't have your best enthusiasm for the mind. Consider why there are major parts of your life that are like this in the first place. How could you meet? What qualities do you like or abhorrence about the relationship? In the event that you list a bigger number of abhorrences than likes, you are more than likely happier without them consuming up valuable space in your life in the first place in any case.

Purchase Less

In the event that you figure out how to purchase less things and toss out what you never again utilize consistently, you will discover the de-jumbling process significantly simpler, also build up a more grounded lined wallet. The less there is to deal with, the less anxiety you will have.

Subtract Dependencies

There are more than lifeless articles that make us subordinate. Individuals, even those that are beneficial for us and our lives, can make us reliant on them for joy. This likewise goes for innovation of various sorts that we as a general public are progressively developing increasingly subject to for accommodation. By decreasing the number of things you have developed reliant on, you are really giving yourself more flexibility to approach your life. This does not mean you need to totally cut these things or people out of your life, however, to decrease your feeling of reliance to these things so that if something somehow managed to happen, your satisfaction and feeling of prosperity isn't all in a couple of egg wicker bin but instead in yourself.

Learn the Importance of Unplugging

We are all guilty of being dependent on our gadgets. Learn the importance of unplugging yourself from your phone, computer, tablet, television, etc. It is best to start in small increments, unplugging a few times a month of in the evening an hour before you go to sleep. This will help with your negative feelings at night and you will fall asleep faster without your phone in your hand in the dark. The major reason to de-plug is so that you can give attention to more important things in your life, like spending some time with family or friends and doing things for yourself that will benefit you far better than liking a few statuses or constantly checking emails.

Stop Comparing

As people, we actually see others and contrast our lives with theirs. Having examinations bobbing all through your mind all the time just prompts an overabundance of stress. Regardless of how incredible you have it, there is continually something that another person has that you need. Figure out how to value you and your life for what it is. Figure out how to acknowledge what you have!

Appreciate the Little Things

The least difficult of delights are the things that light up our lives the most. Regardless of where you are or what conditions you are in, discover something to grin and additionally giggle about. You will feel a programmed arrival of stress on the off chance that you discover something every single day to stay over and be upbeat about. Regardless of whether it is a decent day outside or an infant's chuckle or possesses an aroma similar to a pie heating up, take it in and grin. Life is best comprised of little, yet stupendous minutes.

In my own life, I do my best to grin at every single person that I run over, regardless of whether I know them or they are an aggregate outsider to me. In the event that somebody tried to play out this straightforward and thoroughly free activity to me growing up, my attitude would have been distinctive I am certain. Be the affection that you never got.

Reconsider Your Goals and Priorities

Taking a couple of minutes all the time to truly take a seat and evaluate your life's needs and the objectives you need to accomplish will help you either locate a prosperous way or abandon you stuck in the same ole groove. On the off chance that you persistently continue removing the parts of your life that are essential to you, you will never be fulfilled.

Figure out How to Say NO when it Counts

Actually, we tend to direct fault toward different parts of our lives for making us so worried. In actuality, we are the main ones to fault for feeling along these lines. In the event that you have a desire to live less complex and settled, you should figure out how to state no to individuals and openings that don't suit you. This additionally incorporates letting yourself know no to things that are not among the highest point of that need rundown of yours. It will be distressing to state no at, to begin with, yet it will turn out to be second nature to you. Think about constantly and space for future potential outcomes that will really fuel your objectives!

As you perused in my own story, I was a doormat. I was helping other people however never myself. I generally had others as a primary concern yet never asked myself what I required. You can't pour from any void pot. Meaning, you need to get things done for yourself so as to keep the pot you use to top off the measures of others full and prosperous. Bear in mind the essential individual on the planet is yourself.

Figure out How to Delegate

While saying no is an imperative piece of keeping your life on track and not overwhelming it inside things that you eventually make you unfulfilled, this does not mean it gives you the reason to move in the opposite direction of new open doors or your obligations. Be that as it may, you can figure out how to appoint certain parts of your life. Regardless of whether it is employing another partner to help get past heaps of printed material or instructing your children how to do family unit tasks, appointing some of those duties out to those you trust can enable you to complete things and help with making you feel more expert toward the day's end.

For Your Own Good, Be Timely
We all know how it feels to be rushing around because we woke up late. Learn to get up earlier, leave earlier, etc. Whatever you must do to give yourself time to get to work, school, commitments on time will help you to feel less stress in the long run. It is a good feeling to be early.

Tone Down Multitasking
With all that we are required to complete in a day's opportunity, we have a tendency to overcompensate the procedure of multitasking. Rather, figure out how to separate greater achievements into littler undertakings with the goal that you can appropriately concentrate on those errands that prompt painting the master plan. Figure out how to single-errand!

Unschedule
This runs as an inseparable unit with figuring out how to state no more frequently. It is very superfluous to plan every snapshot of our day to day lives. Figure out how to make more times of open time. This will give you an opportunity to get things done at a pace that you are OK with, prompting a great deal less anxiety.

Back Off

I know this one is substantially harder than it appears. In any case, we as a whole race through life and with regards to the end, we ponder where all that time went. Take in the significance of getting a charge out of time with those you cherish, enjoying sustenance as opposed to scarfing it down.

Help out

While it might appear like making a couple of strides back in the wrong heading to go up against more undertakings, there is no inclination that is as very as awesome as helping another person out. Set aside an opportunity to enable those you to love, volunteer inside your group, assist an elder who looks for help. It is not about being controlling yet rather being merciful when it makes a difference most.

More Grateful Feelings

Building up a disposition of appreciation may not appear like a major stride in improving your life, however, it surely aids the making of positive musings which diminishes stretch definitely. Figure out how to be thankful and acknowledge what you have and of those in your life. In the event that you see life as a blessing, your feeling of bliss will soar.

How to Live in a More Positive Light

With a specific end goal to diminish the pessimism that overrules your life, one must put in the work to improve positive changes and methods for deduction a propensity. There are numerous little changes one can make that can conceivably have altogether positive outcomes in their life. This section is loaded with only a couple of the best ones!

Careful Moving

We are naturally human beings that categorize negative tendencies that have lasting effects on our lives for years to come. All that we do right now is pointed towards a conceivably better standpoint over the long haul. We neglect to set aside the opportunity to appreciate and live in the present. When you invest greater quality energy inside the occasion, it is significantly less demanding to be certain and has practical desires. On the off chance that you invest all your energy, later on, you are simply setting yourself up to be a noteworthy wet blanket. Move moderate amid your morning schedule and whatever is left of your day will ideally be trailed by a similar activity.

Begin Your Day in a Positive Way

The technique in which you begin the day from the earliest starting point sets the tone for the rest of it. This is the reason it's so regularly worried to get up somewhat prior so you can play out your morning schedule at your own pace. We regularly are working at full speed and are vulnerable to losing all sense of direction in push and the loss of energy we have over our lives.

Increase the Value of Another Life

The vibe we convey into the world once a day has an amusing method for returning to embrace us or kick us appropriate in the butt. What you give it normally what you get.

- *Help out* – Lend a hand to a companion when they require it, give somebody a ride, inquire as to whether they require help.

- *Listen* – Learn how to tune in as opposed to talking over individuals. Most circumstances, individuals simply require a listening ear that is non-judging and mindful to what they are stating.

- *Boost temperaments* – Give embraces (when suitable), grin at individuals while looking. Play feel great blocks when hanging out with companions or recommend a moving film. Energize those experiencing intense circumstances.

Try not to Let Fear Overrule Your Life

There will be times you need to take life by the horns, be dangerous and take a risk. Be that as it may, those negative feelings and absence of trust in ourselves has a method for pulling you once again from these open doors. We have a tendency to reach out ambiguous feelings of trepidation to rationalize not taking risks. We are filled with fear rather than what is conceivable on the off chance that we attempt. Ask yourself what is the most noticeably awful that could happen. This will clear a path into making sense of how to invest energy in new circumstances that could prompt conceivably greater turnarounds.

Locate Your Happy Place

Turns out that finding your glad place is a genuine article and is particularly prescribed for those that experience times of tension. Rationally moving when our uneasiness erupts is an extraordinary approach to staying casual, quiet and at the time. It gives us the flexibility to lose ourselves in a specific minute. Bliss is a condition of mind. The more you work on arriving, the less demanding it will move toward becoming for you.

- Recall places that you have been that you have enjoyed for their sights or sounds.

- Use the technique for symbolism or perception to achieve that place you look for.

- Ensure that you pick a place that you encounter upbeat feelings.

- Try to review where you were the point at which those sentiments of profound importance and additionally happiness inundated you.

Maintain liberality

This technique takes a great deal of devoted practice to truly get down. I know over and over I turned out to be more worried and disappointed with attempting to hone contemplation and other such techniques, which made me more on edge. Be that as it may, have confidence in yourself and don't surrender effectively. Trust me, strategies like this are substantially less demanding when said than finished when it comes to disposing of or quieting the negative voices in your psyche. Keep in mind, tolerance is a prudence that is a need now and again. When you get the hang of accomplishing your upbeat place you will need to withdraw there more regularly than you might need to concede and approve!

Compose Written Words from your Inner Self

I know that writing, in general, has helped personal on numerous occasions with regards to my sentiments of cynicism. At whatever point I was feeling especially restless or in some sort of enthusiastic turmoil, I would get a notepad, my telephone or my portable workstation and scribble out my sentiments. Keeping in mind the end goal to do this successfully, let go your dread of judgment. Unless you give your diary or whatever you compose on to another person to peruse, this is only for you to vent. It additionally puts a positive turn on being a sufferer of the tempest of negative feelings that overwhelm one at any given time. I have made numerous extraordinary peruses, for example, short stories and sonnets, from what I was feeling at a specific minute. Try not to consider composing endeavoring to keep away from all the dim things you might be feeling. In fact, you are living at that time by reporting it, as well as over pondering it in a helpful way. Truly, attempt it. I guarantee you that you will feel greatly improved about it. Besides, on the off chance that you compose regularly enough, you may see an example in your life that you wish to or need to change.

Inspiration is a fuel that is exceptionally underestimated. Unless you need to demonstrate your works to another person, you are the special case that can read them. Try not to be dreadful of what you scribble down. It is between you, you're composing utensil and whatever medium you compose upon. Regardless of the possibility that you can't discover the words to depict how you feel, write down graphic words or expressions that may fly up in your mind occasionally. Composing is somewhat similar to work out, particularly in the sense in the event that you are recently beginning. It will feel unusual to compose things that you are considering or compose letters to yourself. Be that as it may, once you get prepared in it, your psyche will ache for composing sessions. Trust me. This is a fundamental way that I figured out how to traverse my youthful years and still keep on practicing when I require a touch of unwinding time or need to loosen up. Composing is not an opportunity to be your own most noticeably awful faultfinder. Unwind, scribble down whatever rings a bell and let the sentencing roll unreservedly.

Discover the Optimism inside Negative Circumstances

I have discovered that a standout amongst the best approaches to make a positive perspective on any sort of circumstance is to pose more accommodating inquiries. What is great about the circumstance? What is another open door that may be existing in it? Thinking like this has a great deal more beneficial outcome on my life than asking what did I do to merit this, and so on. Try not to surge these request, however. Set aside the opportunity to handle your sentiments and musings towards a circumstance. Attempting to compel energy while in enthusiastic turmoil, for the most part, isn't extremely successful.

Develop a Positive Environment

The additional time you spend from outside media, for example, TV, magazines or the World Wide Web, the better. It is basic to have positive impacts throughout your life with a specific end goal to lead your life in such a way. Ask yourself what some negative impacts throughout your life may be and what wellsprings of data prompt negative musings. While experiencing your responses to these requests, consider how you could invest less energy in these things. You now have significant additional time allowed to do things that will have constructive outcomes in your life!

Be Comfortable in Your Own Skin

This one can be a test, particularly for the individuals who are afflicted by the sentiments that they are sufficiently bad and never will be. We fear judgment and attempt to be flawless when in actuality, nobody on this planet can accomplish compulsiveness. Figure out how to acknowledge your identity and the body in which you were conceived in. In the event that you are continually wishing to change things about yourself that are really difficult to transform, you will never be content with yourself. It murders any possibility to be upbeat. When you are not happy with your own particular skin this prompts issues with certainty, confidence and your general prosperity. Separation yourself from individuals who make you feel not as much as cheerful.

Figuring out how to be alright with yourself appears, in any event to me, something that goes back and forth. We as a whole stride foot in circumstances that we withdraw back to our inward middle school self, where we sit ponderously to the side at the center school move. We have a tendency to overlook how far we have come and go to the solace of our shell. In any case, you have to recall that you have come far in your own life and that you have earned the privilege to strut your stuff! In the event that you feel somewhat less sure that what it takes to pull something off, I remain by the platitude 'fake it till you make it!' You can fill a roomful of people with this attitude. It is about having an uplifting point of view toward a circumstance. You should recollect that you are one of a kind and that there is positively nobody out there simply like you. Thus, if not whatever else, be certain about the way that you ought to be more sure with the goal that others can luxuriate in the eminence of your lovely internal hues.

Acknowledge What You Have

In the event that you are continually looking for what others have and what you don't, you will dependably picture your life as the grass is greener in other individuals' yards and not acknowledge and end up plainly appreciative for all the awesome things you have in your life as of now! You will feel always hopeless and as though something is absent. This is simply the same for contrasting with others too. While it might set a specific benchmark to make progress, contrasting yourself as well as other people become unfortunate sooner or later. Ensure your intentions are pointed towards flourishing. Basically, figure out how to acknowledge what you have and set aside the opportunity to recognize that everybody is battling their own fights. You would be shocked by exactly what number of individuals wish they had your life.

Relinquish Anger and Resentment

Hatred towards other individuals is just going to harm you deeply. We hold tight to outrage with the presumption that the individual will, in the long run, acknowledge what they fouled up. In any case, actually, we are just harming ourselves. Figure out how to give up and excuse, regardless of to what extent the procedure takes.

A major piece of me vanquishing negative considerations and feelings was acknowledging and conceding all the developed hatred I had towards those that had treated me terribly previously. Try not to trick yourself into suspecting that you will just need to experience the way toward freeing yourself from irate sentiments just a modest bunch of times throughout your life. It will happen a larger number of times than you need to consider. I have been harmed profoundly by many individuals, which has abandoned me to be attentive and untrusting. I even had developed outrage towards myself from being so careful about the activities of others. In any case, at last, after some time I acknowledged that I am how I am a direct result of all the shitty things I had been through beforehand in my lifetime. Without those awful conditions, I would not be the solid, spurred singular I am today. I have discovered that after some time, the stuff and rubble that originates from the pulverization of our lives can be used to make better forms of ourselves. A spirit that we are glad to claim and live close to. You will realize when you investigate your life that the best parts of you were pulled appropriately from the rubble. Once in a while, it takes putting ourselves out there and associating with others to perceive how significant certain bits of ourselves truly are. Trust me when I say to keep those individuals close and treat them merciful. You will discover them just a few and extremely far between.

Live with an Open Mind

The individuals who are intolerant are just harming themselves. You will feel fomented more so than those that live straightforwardly in view of how immovably you remain in convictions that numerous others may not live by or favor of. In the event that you figure out how to carry on with your life as your own particular and regard that others are more than fit for living theirs as seems to be, you will be more joyful in general.

When I began to see my general surroundings in a great deal more extraordinary and positive light, I picked up a completely new viewpoint of my environment, as well as I figured out how to welcome certain things with more regard. Despite the fact that there were days that persuaded that I didn't have much, once I started to see my reality all the more decidedly, I understood that my life was not all that terrible all things considered. I additionally understood that my negative considerations were something that made me deterred to all the excellent open doors that the world brought to the table me. When you get into this place of acknowledgment you will begin to plunge further into your companionships, connections and even the affinity you have with yourself. It is a warm feeling when you achieve this progression. What's more, one day I trust you do!

Down in the Dumps? Listen to Uplifting Tunes!

There are a lot of studies to demonstrate what effect music has on our brains. On the off chance that you need to be in a perky state of mind, turn up your positive music! It is a certain fire approach to light up your day. Offer it to everyone around you! I know for me specifically getting out and driving for a bit with my music blasted with some of my top picks, cheery tunes cause me to pivot the entire sum of my mindset instantly!

Other Methods to More Positive Living!

- Wake up with the solid held conviction that today will be an awesome day.

- Illuminate those that you adore that you think about them and their prosperity.

- Troubled? Just you have the ability to change your life.

- Things won't generally be awful, intense or harsh. Things will show signs of improvement.

- Make a rundown of the things going appropriately in your life as opposed to harping on every one of the things turning out badly.

- There are dependable individuals that think about you and will tune in, you are never absolutely alone.

- Immerse yourself in your most loved action or interest in the event that you are focused. Anything that lifts your mindset is affirmed!

- Notwithstanding when things don't go your direction or happen out of the blue, figure out how to see things as positive accidents.

- Figure out how to be simple on yourself. Don't generally take a stab at flawlessness.

- Appreciate nature or different spots that assist you escape from reality for a bit. This can be calming and help naturally assuage negative side effects.

- Turn up your main tune. It is a certain fire and snappy approach to liven up!

- Parity your time carefully between work, school, connections and yourself.

- Every day is a blessing. Regard it in that capacity.

- Research has demonstrated that the individuals who are hopeful have a tendency to live more!

- Unplug and step away from anything relative to parts of online networking, schoolwork, and work

- Eat things that support your body. A sound vessel gives a path for more positive energies to be felt for the duration of the day.

- What are you energetic about? Figure out how to wind up noticeably an ace at whatever drives you.

- Satisfactory rest, rest, nourishment, and exercise all assume parts in a sound way of life and psyche.

- Chuckle regularly and grin as much as you can!

Test Negative Thinking

A basic part of discovering alleviation from the tempest of cynicism for those that look for it and will take the necessary steps is figuring out how to provoke your mindset, particularly with regards to reducing negative ways. This section is loaded with approaches in doing only that and hits many spots in all parts of your life!

The most effective method to tolerate uncertainty

As people, we are normally attracted to commonality. We are every one of the somewhat awkward at first in a new environment or around new individuals. In any case, it's essential to open yourself to these sorts of circumstances to expand your perspectives and get your hands on exceptional open doors. Those that live alongside vulnerability tend to need over the top consolation, make a point by point schedules, twofold check things, are not fit for appointing assignments to others and have a tendency to linger.

- *Try to act in an "as though" form* – Write down the things you do to feel increasingly sure about the existence or to evade new circumstances. Look with detail into your regular day to day existence. At that point record practices that can enable you to decrease measures of vulnerability in your life.

- *Practice enduring instability* – Once you have that rundown made, you can begin to hone them, doing as such no less than 3 times each week.

- *Document it* – Keep a record of your activities and how you felt while behaving in them. You will have the capacity to then observe what is working versus what you can eradicate.

Step by step instructions to Solve Daily Life Issues

Every last one of us has issues. We have a tendency keep away from them, when in all actuality overcoming them head on rapidly can prompt a great deal less negative emotions and inconveniences later on. Troublesome issues are a consequence of not having an answer or use of procedures that truly don't work. These can make one be focused and prompt on edge feelings and emotions. These have an impact, by the way, we capacity and feel about ourselves where it counts, regardless of the possibility that we experiment with best to never indicate it outwardly.

- **IS there an issue?** – Come to the acknowledgment if there even is an issue to be settled or not. At that point, it is essential to not disregard it or linger with regards to settling it.

  o *Make a rundown* – Write down issues throughout your life. This will help you to have the capacity to see the issue and approach it in an ideal way.

  o *Use sentiments* – Use negative feelings you have inside you to go to an answer for the issue. What is making you feel along these lines?

  o *Locate the test* – Many circumstances while translating what to do next, we consider ourselves terrible issue solvers. On the off chance that you think along these lines, you will explain nothing. On the off chance that you have issues with associates, for instance, take a shot at relational abilities to determine work-out issues.

- **What is the issue?** – Ask yourself what the circumstance is and what you might want it to be. Are there any snags keeping you from a coveted outcome? Guarantee that you are not expecting things. Get the truths. Figure out how to be particular with regards to characterizing the issue also.

- **Think of arrangements** – Make beyond any doubt to think of more than two or three unique answers for unraveling an issue, just on the off chance that one doesn't wind up working. Figure out how to not pass judgment on your answers before they are even made. Indeed, even the most abnormal of arrangements work adequately! Make out itemized arrangements so that on the off-chance that you should convey them to others, you can do as such easily. Request help when required. There is nothing amiss with have an additional arrangement of hands and another cerebrum to think of arrangements.

Techniques for Relaxation

Meditate

A couple of minutes of training everyday can help ease uneasiness. Research recommends that every day reflection may modify the Cerebrum's neural pathways, making you stronger to stretch.

It's straightforward. Sit up straight with both feet on the floor. Close your eyes. Concentrate your consideration on presenting - so anyone can hear or noiselessly - a positive mantra, for example, "I feel settled" or "I adore myself." Place one hand on your gut to adjust the mantra with your breaths. Give any diverting contemplations a chance to drift by like mists.

Inhale Deeply

Take a 5-minute break and concentrate on your relaxing. Sit up straight, eyes shut, with a hand on your paunch. Gradually breathe in through your nose, feeling the breath begin in your midriff and work its way to the highest point of your head. Turn around the procedure as you breathe out through your mouth.

Be Present

Take 5 minutes and concentrate on just a single conduct with mindfulness. Notice how the air feels all over when you're strolling and how your feet feel hitting the ground. Appreciate the surface and taste of each chomp of sustenance.

When you invest energy at the time and concentrate on your faculties, you should feel less tense.

Connect

Your informal organization is one of your best instruments for taking care of stress. Converse with others - ideally up close and personal, or if nothing else on the telephone. Offer what's happening. You can get a crisp point of view while keeping your association solid.

Get in Tune with your Body

Mentally examine your body to get a feeling of how push influences it every day. Lie on your back, or sit with your feet on the floor. Begin at your toes and work your way up to your scalp, seeing how your body feels.

Conclusion

Thank you for making it through to the end of *Emotional Psychology*.

I trust the substance of this book could enable you to see that even you, yes I am conversing with Negative Nancy in the corner, can develop enough certainty inside yourself to endure forever! While certainty is normally ingrained in a few people, the rest of us must work on ourselves to get a handle on our certainty and not let it sneak past our fingers, regardless of what circumstance we are in.

I trust the data you have recently obtained has given you a liberating sensation, a light toward the finish of a long, unconfident burrow. With a little work and revamping yourself, you can turn out to be similarly as certain as anyone else! You have the ability to be certain; you simply need to locate the correct way that works wonders for you!

That being stated, make certainty and bettered confidence a progressing objective for yourself to accomplish all the time. With a little certainty next to you, you can do anything you set your psyche to! It is about getting up from falling, forgetting about yourself, ignoring your oversights, learning and developing into being a surprisingly better person. As you have learned, certainty is an aptitude that is not actually God given to every one of us. What's more, ever the individuals who are certain don't feel so hot constantly. Now and again, you just got the opportunity to fake it until the point when you make it!

My companions, I wish you fortunes in your adventure of finding the certainty that lives inside yourself. What's more, I trust you discover it with the assistance of this book! Good fortunes!

At long last, on the off chance that you discovered this book helpful in any capacity, an audit on Amazon is constantly valued!